Table Of Contents:

Introduction

As a vegan teen, I wanted to help other teens interested in becoming vegan to achieve their goal. Veganism has become a great movement and it's spreading like wildfire. I have been asked many times by other teens how they should start the transition into veganism. Most teens eventually give up when they try to go vegan. This book will help you succeed and not give up. You can do anything you put your mind to. Many people are curious about the vegan lifestyle, especially teens.

Being vegan has positively changed my life and I want to share the secret of success with you. When I converted to a vegan lifestyle I began feeling better than ever, I also had more energy than ever before. I felt better not only mentally but physically too. Going vegan has given me peace in knowing I am not supporting the abuse and killing of animals.

In this book I will go over how to convince your parents to allow you to vegan, how to have a healthy nutritious diet, how to begin your transition into veganism, and more.

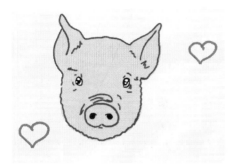

Chapter One
Why Go Vegan?

The main question you need to ask yourself is: Why do you want to go vegan? This is a very important question because if you don't know then you will not likely succeed. This lifestyle takes a lot of self-discipline. What is the point of self-discipline if you don't know why you're doing it? If you don't know why you want to go vegan then take some time to think about what is pushing you towards this lifestyle? Is it animal welfare? Is it for your health? Is it for the environment in general? Think deep and hard about this. Then go online and do some research on these topics. Learn about everything you can and learn your "Why?" In the next few paragraphs I will go over what made me decide to go vegan, and why you should try this lifestyle.

For the Animals

Personally, animal welfare is the main reason I chose to go vegan. After learning about all the cruelty in the animal agriculture industry, I realized that there was no way I could support this industry. Why would I pay someone to directly torture and kill animals? That idea is so absurd. You can't love and eat animals at the same time.

Dairy cows are raped; then when they give birth their babies are taken away immediately. The mother cows then grieve for their calves: any mother could understand the way these cows are feeling. Then the babies are put into isolation and are brutally killed or used in this horrific cycle. There have even been reports of the workers hitting the babies with hammers or kicking them, and even pulling the babies by their ears and tails. If any mothers are reading this, can you imagine this happening to you and your kids? How would you feel if you were in these cows' situations?

Pigs are very smart; they have the intelligence of a three-year-old human child. My point is, that if we measure humanity based on the intelligence of a species, then eating a pig is equivalent to eating a three year old child. Pigs live in horrible conditions on farms. On many pig farms, mother pigs don't even have enough room to turn 360 degrees. When they are nursing their babies, they barely have space to move. The only way they can move is either standing up or laying down. They can't even look at their babies, that's how little space they have. Since pigs are so smart, they know that they are going to die months and even years in advance. That is why people kill them by gas. The pigs fight back, and they scream as they slowly get suffocated.

Chickens are in small cages, to the point where they can't even stretch out their wings. There is no air conditioning in these places, and the chickens get extremely overheated. The chickens are hot, and they can't even cool themselves off. Chickens in the wild only lay around 10 eggs a year, while chickens in this industry lay around 350 eggs a year. This causes them to be extremely deficient in many nutrients. In addition, the chicken's babies get ground up alive if they are males. While the baby girls have to live a horrific life. Can you imagine if this happened to a cat or dog? The outrage people would have. Why do we treat these animals so differently? That is the main reason I went vegan because of all the horrible torture the animals go through for a person's 5 minute benefit.

Health

Another reason people go vegan is for their health. Being vegan has been proven over and over again to be one of the healthiest lifestyles. I'm sure many people are wondering: don't you need to eat meat and dairy to survive? Science has proven over and over again that this is completely false. The reason humans believe that they need meat and dairy to survive is because the agricultural industry has done a great job brainwashing people into believing that you need meat and dairy. How have they done this; you may ask? Through many,

many commercials, and false medical statements. When have you ever seen a commercial about raspberries, strawberries, mangos broccoli, and more? Commercials only advertise hamburgers, hotdogs, and other animal-based products. And these industries use words like "For a man," to make it feel like people need to eat meat. They have been doing this for centuries. In addition to this, they have been paying lobbyists big bucks to convince government officials and agencies to keep quiet about the health problems that are linked to meat and dairy consumption. Nutritionists suggested that doctors should be educated about new studies in nutrition every seven years. However, the agricultural industry was completely against it, so eventually the idea got overturned.

In addition to that, in most medical schools they only teach you about medicine and how to heal with certain medications: students never learn about how to prevent or even heal certain diseases with a plant-based diet. Doctors have not been educated about the way an animal-free diet can help heal diseases. It's no wonder that people believe that you need dairy and meat to live.

Contrary to common belief, eating meat and dairy is not healthy for you and it is definitely not a necessity for life. Animal products are actually causing more deaths in the United States than any other cause of death. Eating meat increases your chance of developing diabetes, heart disease, obesity, cancer, and much more. There has even been a study published in *Cell Metabolism* in March 2014 showing that people who eat a diet that is high in animal proteins from milk, meat and cheese are more likely to die of cancer than someone who eats a plant-based diet. The research also showed the people who ate lots of meat and dairy were more likely to die at an earlier age. Eating meat is almost the same as smoking. There have also been studies showing that people who are vegan live longer and they are much more energized. Eating meat is generally not good for you if you can replace it with something else.

Environment

Another reason people are vegan is for the environment. For example, Greta Thunberg. Though much of the world is focused on transitioning away from fossil fuels as a way to fight climate change, there is another, often-overlooked climate change culprit: animal agriculture and its environmental impact. More than 75% of global warming and greenhouse gasses is caused by animal agriculture. The animals themselves cause 20% of the greenhouse gasses (since animals release methane), furthermore, animal agriculture includes burning down forests to make space for the animals, polluting water, and more: that number jumps to 75%.

"Animal agriculture puts a heavy strain on many of the Earth's finite land, water and energy resources. In order to accommodate the 70 billion animals raised annually for human consumption, a third of the planet's ice-free land surface , as well as nearly sixteen percent of global freshwater , is devoted to growing livestock. Furthermore, a third of worldwide grain production is used to feed livestock. By 2050, the consumption of meat and dairy products is expected to rise 76 and 64 percent respectively , which will increase the resource burden from the industry. Cattle are by far the biggest source of emissions from animal agriculture, with one recent study showing that in an average American diet, beef consumption creates 1,984 pounds of CO_2 annually. Replacing beef with plants would reduce that figure 96 percent, bringing it down to just 73 pounds of CO2e."

Animal Agriculture's Impact on Climate Change." *Climate Nexus* , 23 Apr. 2019, climatenexus.org/climate-issues/food/animal-agricultures-impact-on-climate-cha nge/.

Another reason that people go vegan is actually for other humans. This may not make sense but let me explain. In some countries they grow a lot of food: but they sell it to another country, and they feed that grain to animals that will be killed for meat. The country that sold the food, their own people are starving. The food that is going to animals is actually taken away from starving people. If everyone would be vegan there would no longer be world hunger, because so much of our food goes to feeding livestock. Some people go vegan because they know with less demand for meat more kids will be able to eat.

After listening to all these reasons for why people go vegan, think to yourself: Why do I want to go vegan? Is it for the animals, the starving children, the environment, or your health? After you figure out your "Why," it's time to move on to the next step: dealing with common concerns.

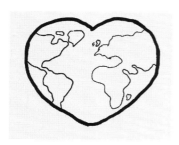

Chapter Two
Counters to Common Concerns

There are plenty of common concerns when it comes to a vegan diet. Most of these concerns have been created over a false prejudice; but at the end of the day they are still there. Some of these concerns might be voiced by your family, yourself, friends, and random people. Here are some common concerns and questions explained.

Is It Hard to Be Vegan?

It's actually easier than you may think! Let's be honest: if you grew up eating eggs, drinking milk, and eating meat at almost every meal, then the idea of going vegan must seems impossible. Most meat-eaters soon learn that the switch is much easier than they think, especially in today's world, when there are so many alternatives.

Where Do You Get Your Protein?

"Despite what you may have heard, protein is actually not much of a worry for most vegans. Not so long ago, conventional wisdom had it that vegans and vegetarians would inevitably develop dangerous protein deficiencies. Over time this myth has largely died out, doubtless due to the fact that have been virtually no instances of vegans dropping dead from lack of protein." (*Vegan.com*)

In perspective, think of the largest land animals. Elephant, cow, giraffe, monkey, horse, ox, etc. Now what do all of these animals eat? All of these HUGE animals eat only greens. Yet they are not protein deficient, they are actually the largest and strongest animals on earth. Think of it like this: you're getting your protein from the same place that the animals you were eating got theirs. You do not have to worry about a protein deficiency. It is always good to make sure you get all your nutrients, however, protein is not something to be worried about, as long as you're eating a wide variety of fruits, vegetables, nuts, and berries. Have you ever seen any vegans drop dead from a protein deficiency? NEVER!

I Only Eat Free-Range Eggs: Is That Okay?

Not if you want to be vegan. Here is why:

"Free-range is certainly better than caged eggs, but virtually every commercial free-range egg farm slaughters its hens. When it comes to animal welfare, free-range eggs are certainly better than battery cage eggs: sometimes even a lot better. But better isn't perfect, and free-range eggs are far from perfect. The hatcheries that provide hens to most free-range egg farms kill their male chicks immediately upon hatching. These newly-hatched male chicks are generally ground up alive; in other cases they smother them in garbage bags or dumpsters. Even if kept in spacious conditions, free-range hens can have an unpleasant life. Like their battery cage counterparts, they've been bred to lay eggs at especially high rates, which in turn exposes them to all manner of health problems. And nearly

all hens, both caged and free-range alike, are slaughtered before reaching the midpoint of their natural lives. That's because egg yields decline as the hens age, and the cost of purchasing new hens is trivial when set against the increased egg output of younger birds. Finally, since cage-free eggs can cost more than twice the price of conventional eggs, there are countless egg farmers who have a big incentive to do the bare minimum possible to label their eggs as cage-free. Unless you personally visit the farm and check the conditions out for yourself, the quality of life for the hens who produce your eggs can fall far short of your expectations." (*Vegan.com*)

Isn't It Expensive to Be Vegan?

Contrary to common belief it is actually much cheaper! Once you learn the basics of a vegan diet, your food bill will be lower than ever. It will be even lower than an omnivorous diet and it will also include better quality food too. There are hundreds even thousands of low-priced, and good quality vegan foods. The key to having a cheap price tag on your food is to not buy vegan junk food. If you go to the grocery store, there are grains, beans, fruits, vegetables, and more. If you buy things by the pound, you can get all sorts of foods for under 50 cents!

"You will dramatically cut costs if you learn when different fruits and vegetables hit peak of season. In North America, that means peas and strawberries in May, cherries in June, peaches and watermelons in August, and apples in November. When you buy produce items at its peak of season, you'll get the highest quality food at the lowest price. If you are extra-motivated to minimize your produce costs, remember that most supermarkets offer outrageously good sale prices on a few produce items every week—just check the market's weekly flyer when you walk into the store." (*Vegan.com*)

I could never be vegan; I like the taste of meat too much!
Just try some of the vegan meats that are on the market today: I promise that you will be impressed. And guess

what is the upside to these vegan meats? They have around the same amount of nutrients and proteins as other meats! Many meat eaters can't even tell the difference between meat and veggie burgers today. There are plenty of meat alternatives that taste exactly the same as meat. Tofu is also an excellent alternative to meat. You can make anything out of tofu, and it tastes delicious. Most Thai restaurants offer tofu as an alternative to meat.

Does the Bible endorse eating animals?

The short answer is No. When it comes to food, the Bible sends many mixed messages. Even with this slight confusion there are still plenty of pro-vegan statements in the Bible. For example in Genesis 1:29 says "And God said: 'Behold, I have given you every **herb** yielding seed, which is upon the face of all the earth, and every **tree** , in which is the fruit of a tree yielding seed—to you it shall be for food." The Old Testament's first book of Daniel also offers a strong statement for a vegan diet. When Daniel and his companions visit the king, Daniel asks permission for the group to eat only vegetables and water for ten days. At the end of this time they're clearly superior health to other guests who ate animal-derived food from the king's table. This shows that the bible also endorses a vegan diet.

Haven't we evolved to eat meat? It's natural!

Actually, eating meat is not very natural. We started eating meat not so long ago. Another interesting thing is that people believe that cavemen were completely carnivorous. Yet that is completely false. The reason people believe this is because they found animal bones at the caveman sites. Yet many scientists have brought up that animal bones will last longer than plant remains. Those same scientists went back to those caveman sites and did some science and they find more plant-based remains than animal-based ones. Another thing to consider is if we were made to be omnivores how come we don't have any omnivore features? If you compare our teeth to omnivores, herbivores, and carnivores teeth, you will see that our teeth resemble a herbivores teeth (Most Herbivores also have canine teeth, similar to our own), our intestines and stomach acid are also almost the exact same as a herbivore. Now look at your nails and teeth, can these things tear and hunt flesh without any tools?

One article said:

"There's no doubt that at many times in history, especially during periods of war and famine, the ability for people to eat meat helped ensure their survival. Likewise, there are some parts of the world today where local populations depend on fish, poultry, or livestock for protein and calories. That's because marginal lands that won't support agriculture can often still support the grazing of livestock, and some coastal areas have insufficient land for farming but access to substantial amounts of fish. That said, few people living in developed countries can credibly claim that their survival depends on animal products. In terms of nutrition, there's nothing in animal products that isn't readily available from a well-planned vegan diet. And if we were really intent on feeding the world, we would stop feeding a huge portion of the worldwide grain crop to livestock (which entails massive food waste), and instead grow grains for human consumption." (Vegan.com)

What would happen to all the animals if we stopped eating them?

If meat consumption declined, fewer animals would be bred into a life of abuse and neglect. It's that simple! Here is a more detailed explanation from an article:

"Wildlife populations would surge, as new habitats were freed up by humankind's smaller dietary foot print. Domesticated cattle and chickens are poorly suited for life in the wild. So in a world that's increasingly vegetarian, we would see their numbers decline with every passing year. Given that most of these domesticated animals suffer incredibly on factory farms, it's probably best for everyone involved if the number of farmed animals raised worldwide falls into steep decline. As fewer farmed animals are raised, much of the land that's currently being used for

pasture or to grow feed crops would revert to nature. So a world with fewer farmed animals would be one with far more wildlife, as well as far more quality habitat for animals currently threatened by human activities..." (*Vegan.com*)

You don't have to kill animals to get dairy and eggs, so what's wrong with those products?

The truth is that all commercially raised animal products include killing.

"When it comes to killing, the only difference from eggs and dairy products is that while meat comes from an animal who *has* been slaughtered, milk and eggs come from animals who *will* be slaughtered. Guaranteed. Every dairy cow and egg-laying hen inevitably goes to slaughter (unless they die prematurely from disease). Milk and eggs have one major thing in common: they're the reproductive products of young females. As cows and chickens age, their milk and egg yields decline markedly. In consequence, nearly all dairy cows and layer hens are sent to slaughter at less than half their natural life expectancy; replaced by younger animals who will also in turn be slaughtered when their yields decline. Add to this that the America's egg industry breeds more than 200 million replacement hens every year, and that it's standard practice for dairy cows to be kept pregnant nine months out of every year. What happens to the males born in these systems? Male chicks are unwanted since, being of the egg-laying variety, they can't profitably be raised for meat. These animals are generally ground up alive, or smothered within hours of hatching. Male calves produced by the dairy industry likewise have little value. Some are sold for a pittance to veal farms, while others are slaughtered immediately upon birth. These dark realities tend to be true regardless of whether we're talking about the worst factory farms, or the best free-range egg farms and organic dairies." (*Vegan.com*)

Cows need to be milked, don't they? We're just doing them a favor?

"Once you understand how the dairy industry operates, you'll see that cows get a raw deal. A cow only needs to be milked because she had her calf taken away from her within a day or two of birth. The calf gets a cheap replacement formula generally made from slaughterhouse plasma and vitamins. Perhaps this strikes you as an unfair deal all the way around. And in a few months, after the cow's milk yields peak, she'll be re-impregnated once again to start the whole cycle all over." (*Vegan.com*)

Don't plants feel pain?

No, plants do not feel pain. They do not have a nervous system, and therefore they cannot feel pain. They were also naturally made to be eaten. Why? You may ask. Well think about it, why would a plant make a fruit with seeds inside? It is hoping an animal will eat it so that it's seeds will spread all over the land. That is the reason why plants taste so good is because many of the plants need animals to eat them and then poop their seeds out. It is how some plants reproduce.

Can you be an athlete on a vegan diet?

This may come as a surprise for many people, but most athletes are vegans. Why? Well, because dairy and meat are not capable of giving them what they need to sustain their active lifestyle. This is well explained in the documentary "The Game Changers" on Netflix.

Don't you need meat to be healthy?

No, you do not need meat to be healthy. Research shows us again and again that a nutritious plant-based diet is beneficial to your health.

If we all went vegan, we'd be overrun with animals?

That is completely false. Farmed animals are not allowed to reproduce naturally. Farmers artificially inseminate them when there is a demand for offspring. As meat and dairy decline in demand, so will the artificial breeding of animals. That means that we will not be overrun by animals. Eventually the few animals that are left, will be set free and find their own place in the ecosystem.

Our teeth/digestive systems are designed for eating meat?

No, they are not. We can digest meat, but our digestive system is different from other carnivorous animals.

"Our guts are longer (so we can digest lots of plant materials) and our teeth are not designed to slice and tear flesh. Our teeth and mouths are the wrong shape to be able to kill and hold captive struggling prey (compare our jaw shape and teeth to a lion — or your pet cat or dog!). That's why humans cook meat before eating it and why we're no good at crunching and munching uncooked bones. As for our sharp teeth, gorillas are entirely vegan — as are almost all primates — and yet have far longer and sharper canine teeth than human beings. The diet of the ancestors of human beings was vegan until they began hunting about one-and-a-half million years ago but even then meat formed just a tiny part of their diet. That's why people live long, healthy lives on vegan diets but would quickly die if they ate nothing but meat." (**Admin**)

Lots of animals kill for food: why shouldn't we?

"Animals do lots of things we don't do and wouldn't do! We shouldn't kill, because we have alternative choices. Lions and tigers have to kill to survive (they are known as obligate carnivores): we don't. Animals can only follow their instincts but we human beings can think about the consequences of our actions. We can recognize the suffering of other animals and we can choose not to inflict it on them. If we choose to make them suffer, what does that say about the human race?" (**Admin**)

Eating meat, fish, eggs and dairy is causing mass pain and suffering; it is destroying the earth and is costing the health services millions of dollars.

It's alright to eat animals if they've had a good life?

"Would it be alright to kill and eat people if they'd had a good life? And what do we mean by a 'good' life, anyway? In the case of animals, we certainly don't mean a long one. 'Meat' animals are killed as babies in the case of lamb and veal calves, or as soon as they become physically mature — the equivalent of human teenagers - and never get to lead any kind of adult life... Animals, of course, want to live just as much as we do. The first instinct every animal has is to survive. By killing them at all, we are taking away from them the most important thing they have; we are denying their intrinsic right to life... It is also naïve to imagine that any farmed animals live good lives: the overwhelming majority of them are exploited, neglected and frustrated on factory farms — forced to live lives of misery by a farming system which sees them only as ways of producing a profit. They then face a violent, frightening death in the slaughterhouse: despite supposedly humane stunning, millions of animals are still conscious when their throats are cut. Even free range and organic animals suffer on farms and they face the same shocking death at a young age as factory-farmed animals" (**Admin**)

How is it okay or even humane to kill an animal that doesn't want to die?

I only eat organic, free-range, fish, chicken, and dairy anyway?

Any choice that people make which reduces an animal suffering is a good choice. Although, why stop at specific kinds of animals. Something that not many people believe is that **Fish** and chicken **feel pain** the same way cows and pigs do. Those animals may seem to be less attractive animals, but that doesn't mean that their lives and suffering are less important to them.

Similarly, although free range and organic animals usually (although not always) live better lives than factory farmed animals, they still suffer in many ways. For example, so-called free-range egg farms may involve thousands of hens being kept in a shed with limited access to outside and to limited land.

Even in the better free range/organic egg farms, all male chicks are killed within hours since they are useless by-products as they do not lay eggs and are too scrawny for meat.

All animals kept for farming are prevented from mixing in normal social groups. Ducks never see their ducklings. Hens never see their chicks. Pigs have their piglets taken away from them at a young age. Dairy cows have their calves ripped from them at one day old. Even on free range farms the male calves are shot (killed) since they don't provide the farm with milk the male cows are the wrong breed for beef. All farms prevent animals from living natural lives. And all are sent for slaughter as soon as there is more profit in killing them than in keeping them alive. Farmers say they love their animals but torturing and killing animals does not sound like love.

There is no need to farm or to slaughter any animal. Eating any kind of meat contributes to animal suffering — and to the environmental and world hunger problems caused by the meat industry. The less meat people eat, the better.

Eating fish doesn't cause suffering?

"Yes, it does. Numerous scientific studies have confirmed that fish do feel pain. Industrial fishing causes them immense suffering because they are killed either by being crushed in the net, having their swim bladders explode when they are brought to the surface or by asphyxiating (being starved of oxygen) on the decks of trawlers. Many fish, especially salmon, are also now intensively farmed and suffer from infectious illnesses, parasites and overcrowding." (**Admin**)

People would lose their jobs if we stopped eating meat.

The vegan food industry is giving more people jobs than dairy, eggs, and meat industries combined. If everyone went vegan, then there would be even more jobs to grow crops for all the people.

I don't mind you being vegan — but you shouldn't try to impose your views on other people. It's a matter of individual choice.

Trying to make people change their minds about going vegan is not imposing your beliefs. The reason vegans try to convince others to change their lifestyle is because one lifestyle (eating animal products) causes death and suffering, while the other lifestyle doesn't. Why wouldn't a vegan try to convince someone else to save the animals, their health, and the environment?

What difference will one person giving up meat make?

A huge difference. By being vegan for one year you save over 400 animals. Can you imagine all those little sad cute faces you ate? By going vegan you can save them from a horrible life.

But we are natural meat eaters?

This is something you will hear a lot as a vegan. That is why I included it in this chapter. "What is the natural human diet? Are humans natural meat-eaters?

Quick test: When you see dead animals on the side of the road, are you tempted to stop and snack on them? Do you daydream about killing cows with your bare hands and eating them raw? If you answered 'no' to these questions, then, like it or not, you're an herbivore. Even though humans take the title of "omnivore" we are anatomically herbivores (our digestive systems and body structures say so).

Humans have short, small, and soft fingernails. Carnivores have sharp and strong nails, called claws, made for tearing meat apart.

Carnivores' jaws move up and down to tear flesh apart and swallow flesh whole. Humans and other herbivores move their jaws from the left to right and they also chew up and down. This allows humans to grind up fruits and vegetables. Like herbivore teeth, humans' back molars are flat made specifically for grinding fibrous plant foods.

Dr. Richard Leakey (a renowned anthropologist) says, "You can't tear flesh by hand, you can't tear hide by hand. Our anterior teeth are not suited for tearing flesh or hide. We don't have large canine teeth, and we wouldn't have been able to deal with food sources that require those large canines."

Stomach acidity is another problem when it comes to human meat eaters. Carnivorous animals swallow their raw flesh whole. They rely on super strong acidic stomach juices to break down flesh and to kill dangerous bacteria: if they didn't have these stomach acids, they would get sick and die. Human stomach acids are much weaker in comparison to a carnivorous animal. Because of this we are unable to digest meat: our stomach acids are made to digest fruits and vegetables. Intestinal length also plays a big role in deciding if we are herbivores.

"Animals who hunt have short intestinal tracts and colons that allow meat to pass through their bodies relatively quickly, before it can rot and cause illness. Humans' intestinal tracts are much longer than those of carnivores of comparable size. Longer intestines allow the body more time to break down fiber and absorb the nutrients from plant-based foods, but they make it dangerous for humans to eat meat. The bacteria in meat have extra time to multiply during the long trip through the digestive system, increasing the risk of food poisoning. Meat actually begins to rot while it makes its way through human intestines, which increases the risk of developing colon cancer." (**peta.org**)

Human Evolution Mistake: If it's so unhealthy or for humans to eat meat, why did our ancestors sometimes turn to animal flesh?

The author of the book *The Power of Your Plate*, Dr. Neal Barnard writes about humans' early food consumption. He explains that we "had diets very much like other great apes, which is to say a largely plant-based diet... Meat-eating probably began by scavenging—eating the leftovers that carnivores had left behind. However, our bodies have never adapted to it. To this day, meat-eaters have a higher incidence of heart disease, cancer, diabetes, and other problems." (peta.org)

"Briana Pobiner, a paleoanthropologist at the Smithsonian's National Museum of Natural History says, "fruit and different plants and other things that we may have eaten maybe became less available. ... The meat-eating that we do, or that our ancestors did even back to the earliest time we were eating meat, is culturally mediated. You need some kind of processing technology in order to eat meat... So, I don't necessarily think we are hardwired to eat meat." (peta.org)

Dairy is also not in our nature. Humans started domesticating cattle about 10,000 years ago. Until then children who stopped breast-feeding stopped producing the enzyme lactase and became lactose intolerant (which is normal). After the domestication of cattle, only certain human groups developed a digestive tract that could digest dairy products. Groups who did not rely on cattle, like the Chinese, Pima tribe, Thai, and the Bantu of West Africa, continue to be lactose intolerant today.

Back in the day only the rich people could afford meat consumption and unsurprisingly, back in the day only the rich were plagued routinely with diseases such as heart disease and obesity. Today meat is accessible for all, so obesity is becoming much more common.

These are some common concerns that you may ask, or someone you know may ask you. Some of these questions you will be asked by people you have just met or even family members. Although some of these questions may seem insane, trust me you will hear them a few times when you start to live this lifestyle.

Chapter Three
Vegan Diet Benefits

The vegan diet may provide health benefits, including:
- Lower cholesterol levels
- Lower blood pressure
- Lower intake of saturated fats
- More vital nutrients
- Lower risk of type 2 diabetes
- Lower risk of heart disease
- Lower risk of certain cancers
- Healthier body weight management

A vegan diet is richer in certain nutrients. Going vegan will make you rely on other foods. Since you eat more of these plant-based foods you will get a higher dose of healthy nutrients.
"For instance, several studies have reported that vegan diets tend to provide more fiber, antioxidants and beneficial plant compounds. They also

appear to be richer in potassium, magnesium, folate and vitamins A, C and E" (Alina)

If you are looking to **lose weight,** a vegan diet will be a great choice. According to a study[1] that show that vegans tend to be thinner and have a lower body mass (BMI). In one study, a vegan diet helped participants lose 9.3 lbs (4.2 kg) more than a control diet over an 18-week study period. Participants on a vegan diet lost more weight than people who followed calorie-restricted diet, even when the vegan groups were allowed to eat until they felt full.

After many studies it shows that vegans have lower blood sugar levels and a vegan diet improves kidney functions. Indeed, vegans tend to have lower blood sugar levels, higher insulin sensitivity and up to a $50 - 78\%$ lower risk of developing type 2 diabetes. Other studies report that diabetics who substitute meat for plant protein may reduce their risk of poor kidney function.

A vegan diet may also protect against certain cancers. According to the World Health Organization, "about one-third of all cancers can be prevented. Vegans generally eat more legumes, fruit and vegetables than non-vegans. This is why a recent study found that vegans have a 15% lower risk of developing or dying from cancer. Vegans also eat more soy products which offer protection against breast cancer. Avoiding animal products also helps reduce the risk of prostate, breast, and colon cancer. Since meats are cooked at such high temperatures, it can promote some other kinds of cancers as well. Vegans also avoid dairy, which many studies show may increase the risk of prostate cancer." (Alina)

[1] Mishra, S, et al. "A Multicenter Randomized Controlled Trial of a Plant-Based Nutrition Program to Reduce Body Weight and Cardiovascular Risk in the Corporate Setting: the GEICO Study." *European Journal of Clinical Nutrition*, Nature Publishing Group, July 2013, www.ncbi.nlm.nih.gov/pubmed/23695207.

Eating a vegan diet lowers the risk of heart disease. "Observational studies comparing vegans to vegetarians and the general population report that vegans may benefit from up to a 75% lower risk of developing high blood pressure... Vegans also have up to a 42% lower risk of dying from heart disease... Since vegans also have lower blood pressure it helps reduce the risk of heart disease. This may be particularly beneficial to heart health since reducing high blood pressure, cholesterol and blood sugar levels may reduce the risk of heart disease by as much as 46%." (Alina)

To make sure you have these health benefits, you will have to make sure you get all of your nutrients: which may not be as hard as it seems.

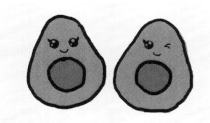

Chapter Four
Getting All Your Nutrients

Although there are all sorts of benefits to being vegan, you must make sure to get all your nutrition. Getting all your nutrients is not going to be as difficult as most people think. You just have to make sure you are eating plenty of grains, berries, fruits, beans, and vegetables. It's best to stay away from the vegan-junk food to have the optimal diet.

Food Group	How Much to Eat
Fruits and Vegetables	At almost every meal and snacks throughout the day

Protein Rich Foods	This includes beans, lentils, chickpeas, tofu, soy, alternatives to milk and yoghurt, and peanuts. This would be recommended for most meals.
Starchy foods	This would be higher fiber foods, such as oats, sweet potato, whole-wheat bread, wholewheat pasta and brown rice. This would be recommended at every meal.
Nuts and seeds (they are very rich in Omega-3 fats)	Some people would recommend having this daily.
Calcium-rich foods	This can include soybeans, broccoli, and kale, plant-based milk, tofu, and more!

Personally, I don't follow this food guideline table to the letter. I just eat what I want, when I want. This is a list of the preferred way you eat as a normal human being. In reality, not many people eat these healthy foods on a daily basis. Being a vegan doesn't mean you eat healthy food all the time. It's up to the person whether they want to be a "healthy vegan" or a "for the animals" vegan.

Many people think that vegans are limited when it comes to food. However, the reality is quite the opposite, vegans are open to all sorts of new food groups and a new way of sustainable living. Just today I bought vegan ice-cream made from coconut milk instead of cow milk! There are a lot of options to choose from.

Of course, it's good to stay healthy, but it's also good to treat yourself. I decided to include my diet and how much I eat, so that you can compare the average teen vegan to the chart.

Food Group	What I eat

Fruits and Vegetables	All the time! I love fruits, I eat them every day: in smoothies, raw, cooked, etc. I eat vegetables every day as well. Who wouldn't? They are delicious! I love having my veggies in a sandwich or soup.
Protein Rich Foods	I have this food all the time. I love lentil soup! So, I usually eat lentil soup at **least** one or two times per week. I also have plant-milk alternatives. I usually put almond milk in my smoothies, and I have coconut milk in some of the ice-cream I buy! Another protein rich food I eat is tofu!

Starchy foods	My favorite food group! Who doesn't love pasta? I have pasta at least a few times a week. I also enjoy whole-wheat bread!
Nuts and seeds (they are very rich in Omega-3 fats)	I eat some sort of nuts every day. For example: sunflower seeds, pistachios, almonds, etc.
Calcium-rich foods	I eat spinach, soymilk, broccoli, and more.

My rule of five is to eat five different varieties of fruits and veggies daily.

Here are some other nutrients tips to keep in mind.

Iron is very important because it plays a key role in the production of red blood cells. Red blood cells help carry oxygen to your body. Iron is found in animals but when you are vegan you no longer eat animals. You can also find iron in dirt, but you're not going to eat dirt. There are plenty of plants that provide the same amount of iron as an animal product. Some of these include beans, broccoli, raisins, wheat, pomegranate, asparagus, tofu, and more. There are also many iron-filled vegan cereals. One tip is to eat a lot of oranges and broccoli because these foods help you digest iron.

Protein : A large myth (as we have gone over before) is that you can only get protein in animal products. That is completely false. First let's go over the function of protein. Protein keeps your skin, bones, muscles, and organs healthy. "Without meat and dairy, you still need to consume essential amino acids. Vegans can get protein from nuts, peanut butter, seeds, grains, and legumes. Non-animal products like tofu and soy milk also provide protein. Vegans have to consider getting enough "complete protein." Protein is made up of small parts called amino acids. These help your metabolism. A complete protein contains all the amino acids your body needs. You can get complete protein by eating certain foods together. Examples include rice and beans, or corn and beans."(Familydoctor.org)

Calcium is commonly found in milk. The milk industry made people believe that milk is the only source of calcium, however, this is just not true. The interesting part is that America is the number one dairy consuming country, yet it is the number one deficient country in calcium intake. This really shows how the dairy industry fooled us. The best ways you can receive calcium is soybeans, broccoli, and kale.

Vitamin D$_3$ helps you absorb calcium. This vitamin also promotes bone growth. Your body produces some vitamin D in response to sunlight. (Interesting fact: most people today are actually deficient in Vitamin D because they don't spend much time outside.) Another way to get vitamin D is by consuming soy-milk, rice milk, and some cereals.

Vitamin B$_{12}$: Ugh. This one. Most vegans have heard people ask about this vitamin. Vegans are actually almost never deficient in this vitamin and actually out of 10 meat eaters at least three of them will be deficient in this vitamin. The reason is because the source of this vitamin is from the dirt. You get vitamin B_{12} from some of the left-over dirt on your produce. Yet since everything is intensely cleaned before you buy it, it's hard to get vitamin B_{12} since there's almost no dirt on your produce. Even the animals that you are eating need a B_{12} supplement, because their food is also intensely cleaned, and it has no left-over dirt. So, in reality the only way to get B_{12} (for meat eaters and vegans) today is either eat a supplement or grow your own food and don't intensely wash it. It's your choice. Just remember that vegans are actually more likely to have B_{12} in their system because they eat more fruits and vegetables, which is more likely to have dirt on it. Make sure to remember this, because everyone you know will ask about this vitamin.

Zinc is vital to your immune system. You can get Zinc in beans, nuts, and soy.

All the vitamins and minerals you need, you can easily receive from a plant-based diet. As a teen vegan you nave a lifetime of good health ahead of you--although this requires making good choices. For example, try not to indulge in too many junk foods. If all you eat is French-fries and soda, then you are not going to live a healthy life. Try to eat quality foods that include all sorts of nutrients and vitamins. Hopefully this chapter helped you know what to keep in mind when being a vegan teen.

Last minute easy tips to remember:
- Eat a rainbow of colorful foods
- Choose high-fiber foods
- Include good sources of protein in most meals
- Eat nuts and seeds daily
- Make sure your diet provides you with iron.
- Get your vitamin D3
- Season food with herbs and spices
- Drink a lot of water
- Keep active

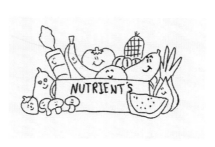

Chapter Five
How to Convince Your Parents?

As a teen vegan you don't live on your own yet, and you most likely don't buy your own food either. That is why you will have to have your parents' permission to go vegan: but in today's world that may still be difficult.

Usually your parents won't let you go vegan, but you have to remember your parents have your best interests at heart. They might not let you go vegan because they are worried about your health. Although this is not very common these days, since many of the vegan myths have been debunked. Sometimes your parents won't let you go vegan because of "tradition." Most of the time, your parents won't let you go vegan because they are misinformed. That is why you need to explain to your parents why you want to go vegan. You need to take their side into consideration. Make sure to stay calm and reasonable, since when you get angry, everyone goes into defense mode and you won't get anywhere. When you're informing your family that you are planning to go vegan, you are going against everything that they have ever believed in about a healthy diet.

You must be well-informed about veganism and should be able to answer simple questions that would help them understand that veganism and safe and nutritious. For example, your parents don't want you to be vegan because they are worried about your health. Well then you should go over how it is completely safe and even better for your health to go vegan. I would recommend going to my nutrition chapter and talk to them about how you can receive all your nutrients from a plant-based diet.

My mom is always convinced with facts that are reasonable and make me healthier. My conversation about veganism transpired as follows:

At a Stop Light in the Car:
Me: "I'm vegan now."
Mom: "Okay."

That was the end of the conversation. Yet that is not going to be the case for everyone. Every family is different: that is why the way you talk about becoming vegan is situational.

I recommend bringing up veganism in a relaxed environment: maybe at dinner, the kitchen table, or while playing a board game. After you have told them about going vegan, they would either completely disagree; be unsure; ask questions; or be completely supportive of your decision.

It's always a bummer when you are super happy with your decision to go vegan, but your parents are a bit iffy about allowing you to make the switch in your diet. We all know it's your parents' job to worry. Guess what: Mom and Dad you don't have to worry at all! Vegan meals provide us with all the nutrients that we need, minus all the saturated fat, cholesterol, and other unhealthy byproducts found in animal flesh, eggs, and dairy foods.

Here's what to tell your parents about going vegan:

It's Healthy!

"Of course, you will need the same amount of nutrients as a vegan as you did when you were still eating meat. Now you will just find them in much healthier places! Have your parents visit the Physicians Committee for Responsible Medicine's website if they have any questions or want to learn how this choice can improve your health and the environment." (*Physicians Committee*)

It's Easy

Go shopping for vegan foods and take your family along. Show them all the vegan options out there. Being a vegan is much easier than it was five, ten, or twenty years ago. I included a shopping guide link in the bibliography of this book that takes you all over the store and helps you find all the vegan foods. Once your parents can see for themselves that there are all sorts of foods ready on the shelves that don't support slaughterhouses and cruelty, they will see that you are not limiting your food range. Soon enough you will all be loving your vegan food too. Trust me, once you buy your vegan groceries you will check the fridge the next day and they are gone: your family has eaten them!

It's Cheap!

Another way to convince your parents to let you go vegan is that being on a vegan diet is really cheap! It's much cheaper than when you ate meat. Your parents will most likely be interested in how they can feed you better foods, for less: so, it's a win-win!

It's Delicious

Another way to convince your parents is to show them that not only you are eating healthier, but you are also eating delicious food! Make a few delicious and healthy vegan foods and share them with your family. After all, the best way to someone's heart is through their stomach. Another upside is most spices are vegan, so you are not changing your culture.

It's Important

Often, the parents' generation doesn't understand the importance of this lifestyle. It's hard for people to understand why someone would go vegan, especially when they don't understand all the cruelty involved. People don't understand what a large impact they are having by buying that cheese, meat or milk. Most people have no idea how horribly animals are treated at factory farms: but that is why you can help them learn. Grab a comfy vegan snack and watch some of these documentaries with your parents and other family members.

Documentaries: "Tyke Elephant Outlaw", "Vegucated", "Vanishing of the Bees", "Forks Over Knives", "Blackfish", "The Beautiful Truth", "Food Matters", "Crazy Sexy Cancer", "Forks Over Knives Presents: The Engine 2 Kitchen Rescue", "Fat, Sick & Nearly Dead", "The Ghosts in Our Machine", "Cowspiracy", "Fast Food Nation", "The Ivory Game", " **What The Health** ", " **The Game Changers** ",

"Live and Let Live", and " Earthlings". You can find most of these documentaries on Netflix and YouTube.

A great documentary that includes no-horrific images of animals in pain is the movie " **The Game Changers** ." It is on Netflix and is easily accessible. It has a lot of very interesting facts and it is a very interesting film--one of my favorites.

Once your parents see what happens to animals, they'll be more likely to understand why you're standing up against something you know is wrong. They might even be proud of you.

Those are some ways to convince your parents. You should have a conversation about why you are going vegan. Address their concerns. Although sometimes, your parents won't budge ...

Chapter 6
If They Still Say No

By not allowing you to be vegan, your parents are forcing you to participate in something horrifying: something that is going to ruin the planet for future generations. It's not right. Nobody should be forced to eat dead bodies if they don't want to. It is always better to have your parents support, since they do buy your food: but at the end of the day, your diet is your choice. Your parents are not you and they can't decide what you will eat. Hopefully it will not come to this, but sometimes it does. Here is how to be vegan even if your parents don't approve.

Get A Job

If you are old enough, you can get a job and buy your own food. You don't have to eat what your parents are giving you if you can eat something else that you bought.

Pick and Choose

If you can't get a job, then you will have to eat your parents food. Your parents don't just buy meat, eggs, and milk, right? They must buy some kind of veggies, fruits, berries, etc. So why not just eat vegan options in your house? For example, it is dinner and you get salad, chicken, and broccoli. Just eat the salad and broccoli. If your parents ask you why you're not eating the chicken just say, "I'm vegan--remember." Although this may make them angry, they will realize that you are serious and that you're not changing your mind. If you do this you have to stay strong to your word. Don't give in. Trust me if you get to this stage, your parents will push back with all of their force, so you have to push back harder.

This chapter is very short because there is not much you can do if your parents aren't supportive. At some point one of you will have to give-in and trust me ... that will be your parents.

Just make sure to show them that you are passionate about being a vegan: show them facts; show them other thriving vegans (there are plenty--many celebrities as well); and make sure to stick to what you want. Stay strong and do what you think is right for the environment, the animals, and your health.

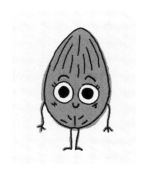

Chapter 7
Beginning the Transition

You've finally decided that you will become vegan. That is when the question comes: Where do I start? Transitioning to a vegan lifestyle can seem really daunting, but often the idea of a big lifestyle change is a lot scarier than actually doing it.

It is important to go at your own pace. If you want to take your time and slowly get rid of one dairy/meat product a week that is fine. If you want to jump straight into a vegan lifestyle that is great too.

Add to Your Diet Before Subtracting from It

It is always good to add something to your diet before you take something away. For example, try a veggie burger (I would recommend Beyond Meat and the

Impossible Burger) before removing burgers from your diet.

Some people want to go all in to be vegan and they won't even try a veggie burger, but some people still love burgers, so it's good to try the vegan alternative. Or you can try tofu: many people dislike tofu, but I would recommend trying to add tofu to a recipe, it can taste really good. Begin replacing dairy milk with milk alternatives such as soy or almond milk.

Before removing something it is good to find an alternative you like that is similar. That way if you crave a certain food, you can improvise with something that is better for your health. Also learn some easy quick meals you can make, so that if you want a quick and nutritious snack you can make it easily. I will include some at the end of this book.

Remember Your Motivation:
I cannot stress this enough: make sure to keep in mind why you are going vegan. If you know why you want to go vegan then you are more likely to

succeed because you have a reason to do it.

Keep A Positive Attitude

Think of the new foods you are trying, and don't think of the foods you are giving up. Say "Yum! This new food is amazing!" and don't say "This is good, but I had to give up meat."

Plan:

If you want to take your time transitioning, I would recommend going in this order: vegetarian, then vegan. Or, vegetarian; then no more fried/boiled eggs; then no more raw milk; then no more cheese; then no more bakery items with dairy; then no ice-cream; then fully vegan.

Try to keep to your plan: because if you don't go with your plan, you might lose your passion to keep up with going vegan. You will be like, "I ate one ice-cream, what is one more?"

You can also jump straight into veganism. I think this might be difficult, but it can also be thought of as a challenge. If you like challenges then I would recommend jumping straight into veganism. You will feel very empowered by doing so.

Do whichever one is the best for you.

Veganize Your Favorite Meals

This one is important. We all have favorite meals, but most of those meals include meat or dairy. So, I would recommend veganizing your meals. Here is an example:

Pizza -> Vegan Pizza (I would recommend just getting a pizza without cheese. Pizza without cheese is actually better than pizza with cheese, if you add some basil. Yum! Just make pizza without cheese! Add any toppings you want! Trust me it's really good! Just try it!)

Make Vegan Food Always Available to You

Since your family isn't vegan, there will always be temptations: that is why you always need to have vegan snacks and meals laying around the house.

Make Sure to Get All Your Nutrients

Make sure to get all your nutrients. This is very easy to do, but try to eat a variety of vegetables, fruits, berries, etc.

A Summary on how to transition into veganism

- Transition at your own time, but don't procrastinate.

- Try starting with easy foods.

- Have fun with it by trying new foods!

- Veganize Your Favorite Meals

- Make sure to stock your kitchen to always have vegan foods available

- Try meal planning: it is very fun!

- Don't over-complicate things (it's really not that hard)

- Try to find a support system (even if your family won't support you,

try to find people who will)

In conclusion, just remember to have a why mindset, to expand your knowledge, go vegetarian first, add foods before subtracting foods, veganize your favorite meals, stock up on vegan food options, be prepared, go at your own pace, and try to find a support group (try Instagram, there are a lot of great vegan groups on there).

That is how to start a transition into veganism. There is also a bunch of information on how to transition into veganism online. Make sure to stay healthy.

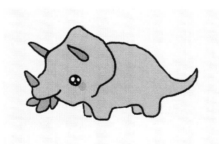

Chapter 8
Things to Watch Out For

As a vegan you will have to watch out for ingredients in the products and you will need to read the back of a lot of product labels (a.k.a. the ingredients). Something might seem vegan, but there are some **keywords** to look out for. This chapter will go over certain words on the ingredient label that means something isn't vegan. Here are some things to look out for that could be in foods or supplements.

Carmine / cochineal is a food coloring that is made out of crushed beetles. So, it's not vegan. I know gross--who crushes a bug and eats it?

Shellac : This is a glaze that is made out of beetles (female scale insects Tachardia lacca). It is commonly found in hard candies and sprinkles (yuck!)

Casein : this is a milk product that is sometimes found in protein shakes.

Whey : This is a dairy product and it is used as an additive in a wide variety of foods.

Lactose is made from milk; it is a sugar.

Collagen is made from the skin, bones, and connective tissues of animals such as cows, chickens, pigs, and fish. It is mainly used in cosmetics

Elastin is found in the neck ligaments and aorta of bovine, similar to collagen.

Keratin is made from the skin, bones, and connective tissues of animals such as cows, chickens, pigs, and fish.

Aspic is an industry alternative to gelatin. It is made from clarified meat, fish or vegetable stocks and gelatin.

Gelatin is made of melted bones and it is mainly used in candy.

Lard / tallow is made of animal fat.

Honey is food for bees, made by bees (technically as a vegan you are not supposed to have honey, although some vegans do have honey and they do not consider it to be bad).

Propolis is used by bees in the construction of their hives. This can be used in all sorts of products.

Royal Jelly is the secretion of the throat gland of the honeybee.

Vitamin D3 is made from fish-liver oil. It is found in creams, lotions and other cosmetics.

Albumen / albumin is made from eggs (most of the time; but it's better not to risk it).

Isinglass is a substance made from the dried bladders of fish. It is mainly used for the clarification of wine and beer.

Cod liver oil is used in a lot of vitamins and supplements. **Pepsin** is made from the stomachs of pigs. It is a clotting agent used in vitamins.

Natural Flavors does not necessarily mean the product is vegan, but I wouldn't worry about that too much, just make sure to check the whole label. In some countries food additives made from insects have to be referred to as 'E Numbers.' An example would be E120.

'May Contain' Labeling

If something says, "May contain eggs or milk." This product may still be considered vegan. When it says, "may contain," it means that this product was manufactured in a building that also manufactures products that include milk and eggs.

Dairy-free and lactose-free are completely different things. Lactose-free is just getting rid of the product in milk that makes lactose-intolerant people unable to digest milk. Dairy-free means that the product doesn't include milk: so just make sure to check the ingredients list.

There will always be moments where you are unsure if something is vegan. On all products there should be a contact or service number. If you want to make sure something is vegan, all you have to do is call that number and ask.

At the end of the day all you have to do is read the ingredients list and watch out for the keywords I listed above.

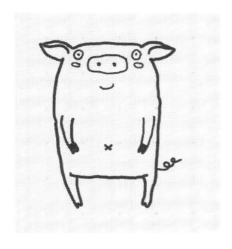

Chapter 9
Eating Out & Breaking Down Menus

Eating out may not be as difficult as you think: but you will have to learn to manage the menu. For example: Let's say a menu offers pizza. Why not ask for the pizza to not have cheese? Trust me, it's better than you think. Going to a burger place? Ask about their veggie burgers. Ask about their French-fries, that is an option for something to eat. Just make sure to check what the fries are cooked in, sometimes French-fries are cooked in beef fat. There are so many ways to get vegan options at a restaurant. If you want a salad but most salads come with cheese, you can ask for a salad without cheese or you can ask them to switch to cheese for something else like avocado.

If you are going out with friends, and if you know that a restaurant has no vegan options, why not bring your own meal? It's honestly really fun!

Many restaurants identify vegetarian and vegan meals with a little green leaf on the menu.

Many Thai places provide vegan options. Sushi places also have vegan sushi, which is really tasty! Many donut places also provide vegan donuts! (Whole foods has great vegan donuts) There are some really great cupcake stores that provide vegan cupcakes! My favorite vegan cupcake store is "Yummy Cupcakes!"

You just need to explore where you live and find all the awesome vegan foods! Those are some ways to navigate a menu.

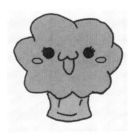

Chapter 10
Dealing with Judgment

Get ready for judgment! Trust me, people judge. A lot less people judge today because the newer generation is definitely more up to date about veganism.

After becoming vegan you are usually upset at the thought of meat and dairy. You look at the people around you and think why are these people using animal products? It's killing the environment, the animals, their health, and more. Remember that is not your problem, so try to keep out of people's way. You can try to educate them, but you can't change them.

Yet as a vegan teen, animal products most likely surround your everyday life. Trust me you're going to hate it: yet at some point you just have to understand that you can't control it. You can only control yourself.

This chapter is about judgment. A keyway to deal with judgment is to be educated. Trust me, lots of people think they are doctors the minute they find out that you are vegan. "What about yourB$_{12}$? "Those people don't even know what B$_{12}$ is: that is why you need to stay educated.

Go to my nutrition chapter and learn more by doing research and talking to your local physician. Once you know what you are doing and you know the facts, it's not that difficult to deal with judgment--because at the end of the day it's your decision. Make sure to own it.

Be confident

"If you know what you are good at, you're less likely to be affected by what others say or think about you. Be confident in your abilities and know your own shortcomings better than anyone else. If someone has something to say about you based on what they think, what does that really have to do with you?

Your Inner Critic!

That little voice in your head can get pretty loud. Recognizing your inner critic and any negative thoughts that creep up on you is the first step in overcoming fear, self-sabotage and self-doubt.

Be Yourself, Trust Yourself

Allowing someone else's judgment to cloud your own perception of yourself makes them a priority and gives them power in your life. If you tend to do this, knock it off. You are the expert on your life. You know yourself better than anyone. You have to trust yourself and your abilities." (**Andrea**)

There is not much advice I can give, just that there is going to be some judgment. The only way you can avoid the effects of judgment is by staying strong, staying educated, and believing in yourself.

Chapter 11
Recipes

To be successful at becoming a vegan you will need some quick and easy recipes so that you don't go back to wanting a quick and easy animal meal. This chapter will be full of delicious, super easy and healthy vegan recipes! Remember that before you go vegan, you need to find meals that you really enjoy. Find alternatives to animal products that you used to like.

Rice Noodle Arugula

This recipe is absolutely delicious, and it takes less than two minutes to make! This is one of my favorites to-go meals!

All you need:
- Thin rice noodles - Arugula

Recommendations
- Green beans
- Any left-over vegetables you have!

Instructions:
1. Boil some water
2. Place rice noodles in a bowl with any other vegetables 3. Let the rice noodles sit for around 30 seconds.
4. Drain the water
5. Add arugula
6. And you're done!

Burrito Bowl:

This is a quick and easy meal that should take no more than five minutes! It is also easily customizable to your tastes!

You will Need:
- Pre-cooked Brown or white Rice - Beans of your choice
- Some lettuce or spinach

Recommendations: - Tomatoes
- Corn
- Tofu

- Other veggies - Cilantro
- Salt
- Pepper

- Chili Pepper
- Cumin
- Smoked Chipotle pepper

Instructions:
1. Pre-cook the rice (have it ready beforehand)
2. Cook black beans or use canned beans (warm them up)
3. Put the rice, beans, lettuce, and other veggies in a bowl. 4. Mix
5. Then EAT!! It's easy as that!

Pasta :

I feel like most people know how to make pasta! And yes,

most pasta is vegan! Just make sure to check the packaging. You can also add some tomato because most tomato sauce is also vegan!

You will need: - Pasta

Recommended:
- Tomato sauce

Instructions:
- Boil water
- Add salt and pepper
- Add pasta
- Cook for however long pasta packaging says too - Drain water
- Put pasta on plate
- Add olive oil and maybe basil leaf (for flavor)

Tomato Sauce
- Put sauce in pot
- Don't forget to put a lid over the tomato sauce - Cook till boiling
- Pour over pasta

Falafel

I personally just buy a frozen falafel and put it in the oven for 5-15 minutes. If you go to a restaurant that has falafel, I would recommend to try them because they are honestly delicious.

You will need:
- Frozen falafel

Recommended:
- Ketchup (Personally I don't like ketchup, but many people do) - Spinach (It's a good side dish)

Instructions: Read the back of the falafel package to know how to cook them. Usually you just bake them for a few minutes!

Chia Pudding

Chia pudding is one of the healthiest breakfasts (or snack) you can eat. It is also pretty tasty.

You will Need:
- Chia seeds
- Almond milk (or nut milk of your choice) - Maple syrup

Recommended:
- Berries - Jam

Instructions :
All you do is put the chia seeds, vegan-milk, and sweetener in a bowl. Then just mix them all together. Leave it in the fridge overnight. Then you have a quick and easy pudding to eat throughout the day.

Pizza

Oh my gosh, this is so good you can't even imagine!

All you will need:

- Pizza dough (make sure it's vegan)

- Tomato sauce

- Vegan Cheese (Optional)

Recommended Toppings: - Mushrooms
- Olives
- Fresh basil

- Onions
- Peppers
- Any of your - You can add

Instructions:
other favorite toppings.
vegan cheese, but I wouldn't recommend it
1. Preheat oven to 400-425 degrees 2. Make pizza dough in a round shape 3. Put sauce on pizza dough
4. Add toppings
5. Put in oven for 5-15 minutes.

Vegan Lasagna

Now this may take longer to make, but you can eat it throughout the week: it reheats really well!

Ingredients:
- 1 box lasagna noodles (for people who want to put in minimal effort [a.k.a., me] get oven-ready lasagna noodles. Make sure to check the lasagna-noodle packaging: some lasagna noodles aren't vegan.)

- 1 cup of packaged tofu, drained. This is optional, but it does add more texture and protein.
- Some salt
- Some pepper

- 1 tbsp. olive oil
- 1 onion
- 3 garlic cloves
- 2 tsp. dried oregano
- Package of mushrooms, sliced (Optional)
- 2 cups of spinach (Optional)
- Marinara sauce

FOR THE WHITE TOMATO SAUCE
- 1/4 c. olive oil
- 1/4 c. all-purpose

- flour 2 1/2 c.
- Almond milk (or other non-dairy milk)
- 2 tbsp. nutritional yeast (Optional)
- 1/2 tsp. garlic powder
- salt
- Freshly ground black pepper
- 2 c. marinara sauce
- 3 tomatoes thinly sliced
- 1/4 c. thinly sliced basil

Directions :

1. Preheat the oven to 350oF.
2. Boil lasagna noodles (if not oven-bake ready lasagna

noodles).
3. Wrap tofu in cloth, then press out as much liquid as

possible. Once it is well drained, crumble with two forks and then season it with salt and pepper. Then, set it aside.

4. In a frying pan heat oil, add onion, garlic, and season with salt, pepper, and 1 tsp oregano. After a few minutes add mushrooms and cook until the mushrooms have softened. Then add spinach and mix in the pan until

completely combined. Then remove from heat and set aside.

5. Now it is time to make the white sauce. Add olive oil, then add flour and whisk to combine the two. Cook until it is lightly golden and nutty (1 to 2 minutes). Whisk in any kind of vegan milk. Stir in nutritional yeast (optional) then add garlic powder and season with salt and pepper. Bring to a simmer and let cook until thickened (8 to 10 minutes.)

6.Now it is time to build the lasagna! In a large baking dish, spoon 1⁄4 cup marinara sauce onto each layer of

noodles. Top with an even layer of vegetable mixture, tofu, marinara sauce, and white sauce. Repeat until all ingredients are used, ending in marinara. Then season with salt, pepper and remaining oregano.

7.Then put it in the oven and bake it for 35-40 minutes, until tomatoes are cooked, and lasagna is heated through. Then remove from oven and garnish with basil. Then eat it!

Fried or Boiled Corn

Corn is super good! Like, who doesn't love corn?

Ingredients: - Corn
- Salt

- Pepper (Optional)

Recommended:
- Some spices

Instructions:
1. Boil water
2. Add salt
3. Add corn
4. Let boil for 5-15 minutes

1. Turn on grill
2. Put corn on grill
3. Cook for 5-15 minutes 4. Eat up!

Veggie Burger:

If you're going vegan for the animals, and you still crave that juicy burger, here is a veggie burger that tastes just like meat. Remember, I am showing you the easiest recipes, so this will be a store-bought patty.

Ingredients:
- Impossible meat or Beyond Meat - Lettuce
- Bun
- Any other toppings you like

Instructions:
1. If Impossible meat, shape it into a flat cylinder 2. Place on grill or frying pan
3. Once done cooking, place vegan-meat in bun
4. Add toppings like lettuce
5. Eat finished vegan burger

Quinoa Salad

Quinoa Salad is so good! There are hundreds of different ways to make quinoa salad. This is just the easiest way, for a quick meal!

Ingredients

For the Dressing:

- 1/4 cup olive oil
- 1 clove minced garlic
- 2 tablespoons lemon juice from 1 large lemon
- 1 tablespoon golden balsamic vinegar or champagne vinegar
- 1 teaspoon pure maple syrup or agave nectar
- Kosher salt and black pepper to taste

For the Salad:

- 2 cups cooked quinoa
- 2 cups fresh spinach leaves, chopped
- 1 cup chopped cucumber
- 1 cup halved grape or cherry tomatoes
- 1 large avocado pitted, peeled, and chopped
- 2 green onions sliced

- Kosher salt and black pepper to taste

Instructions :

1. Make the dressing. In a small bowl or jar, whisk together the olive oil, garlic, lemon juice, vinegar, maple syrup or honey, salt and pepper. Set aside.

2. In a large bowl, combine cooked quinoa (cold), spinach, cucumber, tomatoes, avocado, and green onions.

3. Drizzle salad with dressing and gently stir until salad is coated with the dressing. Season with salt and pepper, to taste. Serve.

Lentil Soup

I love lentil soup--it's so good and refreshing! If you haven't had lentil soup you better try some!

Ingredients :
1 onion, chopped

1/4 cup olive oil
2 carrots, diced
2 stalks celery, chopped
2 cloves garlic, minced
1 teaspoon dried oregano
1 bay leaf
1 teaspoon dried basil
1 (14.5 ounce) can crushed tomatoes
2 cups dry lentils
8 cups water
1/2 cup spinach, rinsed and thinly sliced
2 tablespoons vinegar
salt to taste
ground black pepper to taste

Instructions:
Add everything to soup, let cook for about 40 minutes.

Those are some quick and easy recipes that don't take that much time and ingredients to make. I hope at least one of these recipes sound tasty. These are some of my favorite recipes as well, so it's not just off the internet stuff, I have actually made these in my everyday life!

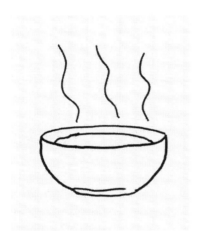

Chapter 12
Conclusion

This is the last chapter of this guide on how to be a vegan teen. It will be difficult at first, I won't lie: but it's not as difficult as most people assume. Although your family may not be vegan, at least you are--and that says a lot about your character.

If your family doesn't want you to be vegan just remember that it's your body and your choice. Even though your family created you, it doesn't mean they own you. You can make your own decisions for your body. Do not let your body become a graveyard of animals.

There are hundreds of reasons to going vegan. Almost every world problem can be linked to eating meat, no joke. World hunger? All the food is going to the animals. If the world went plant-based, that food would go to people. If everyone went vegan, world hunger wouldn't exist. Global warming? The main cause for global warming is cow flatulence. If one person stopped eating meat, dairy, and eggs, that would be almost equivalent to no longer driving 50 million cars. Just eating one vegan meal a day is equal to taking 16 million cars off the roads.

Veganism is also a great way to fight many illnesses like diabetes and heart disease. There is scientific evidence that supports this claim.

Many athletes are changing to a plant-based diet because it's better for the body to function on plants than on meat. Just watch the documentary "The Game Changers" to learn more.

There are hundreds of delicious vegan recipes! If you eat something with eggs, dairy, or meat, I promise you there's a vegan alternative! Make sure to have some quick and easy vegan recipes while you are becoming vegan.

Beginning the transition isn't that difficult. Just slowly cut out animal products. I would recommend starting with milk products, then egg products, and last meat products. Make each change every week. Start with the first week of no more milk; the second week no more eggs; then the last week no more meat: but you can do this in any order that you please. I started with no meat, and then I just cut out other animal products. Just take your time, but don't come to a standstill.

Getting all your nutrients is also very important: make sure to keep that in mind. Eat a lot of grains, beans, nuts, vegetables, berries and fruits. You can of course eat vegan junk food like vegan cupcakes, vegan cheese, vegan ice cream, vegan meat, etc.: but if you want to get all your nutrients, you better stick to some whole foods.

There are a lot of things on labels to watch out for as a vegan. If you don't know if something is vegan, check the label; and if you don't know if an ingredient is vegan then look that ingredient up, and figure out what it is. You can also always call the supplier using the phone number on the product.

Eating at restaurants isn't very difficult: you just need to learn how to manage the menu. You need to learn how to ask them to replace an animal product with a vegan product. For example, want a salad? Just ask, "Can I have the salad without cheese?" the waiter will most likely say "yes." Or you can ask "Can I have the salad but replace the cheese with avocado." That is just one way to manage the menu.

Although it may seem difficult, it really isn't. It is a lot of trial and error, but at the end of the day, you are strong and you're doing an amazing thing.

Just buying this book says that you have an interest in bettering the world, and I applaud you for it. Just trying to go vegan makes such a large positive impact on this world. Although you may have to face some criticism, remember that you are strong, and that you are doing what's right.

Bibliography :

- Answers to Common Vegan Questions. Vegan.com, www.vegan.com/answers/ .
- Animal Agriculture's Impact on Climate Change." Climate Nexus, 23 Apr. 2019, climatenexus.org/climate-issues/food/animal-agricultures-impact -on-climate-change/

- Admin. "Top 20 Questions about Veganism." Viva! - The Vegan Charity , 5 Sept. 2019, www.viva.org.uk/going-vegetarian-vegan/going-veggie/how/20-ques tions.
- Petre, Alina. "6 Science-Based Health Benefits of Eating Vegan." Healthline, Healthline Media, 23 Sept. 2016, www.healthline.com/nutrition/vegan-diet-benefits#section1.
- Staff, Familydoctor.org Editorial. "Vegan Diet: How to Get the Nutrients You Need." Familydoctor.org, 14 July 2017, familydoctor.org/vegan-diet-how-to-get-the-nutrients-you-need/.
- Staff, Familydoctor.org Editorial. "Vegan Diet: How to Get the Nutrients You Need." Familydoctor.org, 14 July 2017, familydoctor.org/vegan-diet-how-to-get-the-nutrients-you-need/.
- "Vegan Label Reading Guide." Veganuary , veganuary.com/starter-kit/vegan-label-reading-guide/.
- "Here Are the Real Facts About Humans and Meat." PETA, 23 Jan. 2018, www.peta.org/living/food/really-natural-truth-humans-eating-mea t/.
- "Health Topics." Physicians Committee for Responsible Medicine, www.pcrm.org/health-topics.
- "Guide to Vegan Grocery Shopping." peta2, www.peta2.com/vegan-life/guide-to-vegan-grocery-shopping/.
- "13 Movies on Netflix That'll Move You to Change the World." peta2, 2 Apr. 2017, www.peta2.com/news/animal-rights-movies-netflix/.

- Schroll, Andrea. "5 Ways To Overcome Fear Of Judgment." HuffPost , HuffPost, 14 June 2017, www.huffpost.com/entry/5-ways-to-overcome-fear-of-judgment_b_1039 6254.

One of Athena's Published Articles on Veganism

A Plant-Based Diet

To many Americans, eating an omnivore diet is a common practice. In fact, a whopping 99.5% of Americans eat an omnivore diet. Recently, eating a plant based diet (Vegan) has become a trend in America. This trend has opened the doors for humans, animals, and the environment alike. This lifestyle has also become much more affordable, efficient, and rewarding. Being vegan has become so much easier than it was a few years ago. Today you have hundreds of plant-based companies such as Impossible Burgers, Beyond Meat, Gardein, Daiya Foods, Tofurky, and so many more. Most important, studies suggest that eating a plant based diet helps prevent heart disease, antibiotic resistance, cardiovascular disease, high blood pressure, high cholesterol, Type 2 diabetes, Breast cancer, colon cancer, prostate cancer, and more. There are even some studies that show that a plant based diet can delay Alzheimer's disease and dementia.

Eating a plant-based diet can prevent many diseases and health problems for any reasons. A British study indicates that a plant-based diet reduces the risk of heart disease and type 2 diabetes. The study even goes as far as to show that a plant-based diet can prevent strokes and heart attacks. [1] because in animal products there are a lot of saturated fats and cholesterol. When you cut animal products out of your diet those unhealthy substances no longer have the ability to clog your arteries. Another major study showed that men with prostate cancer who changed their diet from omnivore to herbivore, had their prostate cancer either stop progressing or reversing the illness all together. Another major disease that is prevented by a plant based diet is breast cancer. In countries where women eat very little animal products, there is a much lower chance of getting breast cancer. Antibiotic resistance is also becoming a huge deal and the main cause of antibiotic resistance is a meat based diet. Animals for consumption are treated so poorly they are pumped with antibiotics to keep them alive. As people eat those animal consumed antibiotics they slowly become more and more resistant causing a lot of problems for the human health.

After people educated on eating a plant-based diet that prevent certain diseases, a few questions come to mind; If we weren't meant to eat animal products, how come our ancestors did? The answer is; they didn't! Our ancestors were completely herbivorous. Did you know that the strongest roman fighters (gladiators) where all vegan? They ate a plant based diet because it was the healthiest way to get all their nutrients and to stay strong. They had the right idea all along. After knowing that our ancestors didn't eat meat you may ask "then how come they started eating meat?" Honestly it was dire circumstances. Humans couldn't find any food and they began eating other animals. "What about our canines?" the answer to that question is all herbivores have canines. Now look at your "canines" and think can they tear raw skin, flesh, and bone apart with one bite? Of course not, those canines are made for gripping and ripping plants!

Another interesting thing to think deeper about is that we have to cook our meat, would you even dare to eat raw beef or chicken? When you see a squirrel do you ever feel like getting on the ground and chancing it around (without any weapons) for food? Do you want to tear that squirrel apart with your teeth and fingernails? Another interesting thing to think of is cow milk. A lot of people believe it is a necessity for calcium. Let's put that into perspective, America is the number one dairy consumer, and yet it is the most calcium deficient country. No other animal drinks other animals milk. It just unnatural, that is why more than half the population is lactose intolerant. It's actually a genetic mutation to be able to be able to even digest milk. Most studies even show that "healthy meat" like chicken, is not as healthy as we think it is. Chicken is basically the same thing as red-meat. A few studies published showed that people who ate red meat and people who ate white meat both had a higher chance of having a chemical called TMAO, and this chemical is linked to causing heart disease. Another common question is about B12.

Interesting enough B12 is actually found in dirt. The only way you get B12 from animals is from the B12 supplements that the animals are receiving. One out of every three Americans (meat eaters included) are B12 deficient because our food is cleaned so intensely with pesticides. In the modern world, the best way to get your B12 vitamin (for meat-eaters as well) is through a supplement. Another question arises is there enough un-forested land to feed everyone on a plant-based diet? Actually 75% of out plant-based food is used to feed animals we eat. If people stopped eating animals, and just ate plants we could feed the entire world's population twice with the current plant-based food we produce for animals and humans. If everyone went vegan there would be no more world hunger, assuming equitable distribution of food around the world. A lot of poor countries actually sell their grain to animal farms, while there own population of children starve, just so that the rich people can have their meat. The final question is if everyone went vegan what will happen to the animals used for food? Well the animals will be just fine. Animals are forcibly bread as supply to satisfy demand. As demand decreases so will the forced breeding and herds would stabilize.

A plant based diet is undeniably beneficial for your health, the environment, and the animals. At the end of the day, think more deeply about what you are eating. Put your "common knowledge" into perspective. Is what your saying and doing making sense? Are you truly eating what is necessary or even healthy for your body? What still remains a mystery is why people are still eating animal based products when they are causing some of the biggest health problems in the world.

1. Tuso, Philip J, et al. "Nutritional Update for Physicians: Plant-Based Diets." *The Permanente Journal*, The Permanente Journal, 2013, www.ncbi.nlm.nih.gov/pmc/articles/PMC3662288/ .

2. Louie Psihoyos, The Game Changers, James Cameron Arnold Schwarzenegger Jackie Chan Lewis Hamilton Novak Djokovic Chris Paul Joseph Pace James Wilks, Joseph Pace Mark Monroe Shannon Kornelsen Starring James Wilks Arnold Schwarzenegger Lewis Hamilton Patrik Baboumian, September 16, 2019.

About The Author: Athena M. Johnson

Athena M. Johnson is a 14 year old college student. She went vegan in 2019 and wanted to share her experience with other teens wanting to go vegan. As an animal rights activist she knows that animal rights matter, and that cruelty has no place in our society.

Check Out Athena's Blog:

http://athena909180359.wordpress.com

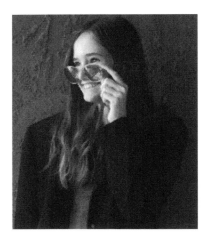